Meal planning for diabetics

Food recipes to stay healthy when diagnosed with diabetes

Amanda J. Eric

Table of contents

Chapter I

- **What is diabetes**
- **Types of diabetes**

What is diabetes all about?

Diabetes mellitus, sometimes known as just diabetes, is a metabolic condition that raises blood sugar levels.

Insulin is a hormone that transports sugar from the blood into your cells where it may be stored or utilized as fuel. When you have diabetes, your body can't utilize the insulin it does manufacture or doesn't produce enough of it.

Diabetes-related high blood sugar left untreated may harm your kidneys, nerves, eyes, and other organs. However, you can safeguard your health by learning about diabetes and taking measures to avoid or control it.

Despite having a similar name to diabetes mellitus, the uncommon illness known as diabetes insipidus is unrelated. Your kidneys are removed from your body too much fluid in a separate ailment.

Each kind of diabetes has specific symptoms, underlying conditions, and therapies.

Find out more about the differences between these categories.

Prediabetes

When your blood sugar is higher than normal but not high enough to be diagnosed with type 2 diabetes, the condition is known as prediabetes. It happens when your body's cells don't react to insulin as they should. Later on, type 2 diabetes may result from this.

According to experts, more than one-third of Americans have prediabetes, yet more than 80%

of those individuals are completely unaware of their condition.

The signs of diabetes

The onset of diabetes is accompanied by increases in blood sugar.

General signs

Diabetes's typical signs and symptoms include:

Increased appetite
More hunger for food weight loss
Urinary frequency hazy vision
Severe exhaustion
Not-healing wounds

The signs in males

Men with diabetes may exhibit the following symptoms in addition to The common ones:

A diminished lust for life
Erection problems (ED)
Weak muscle power

Signs in women

Diabetes in women may cause symptoms like:

Vulvar aridity
Infections of the urinary tract
Candida infections
Itching, dry skin

The conclusion

Diabetes symptoms might be so subtle that they are first difficult to identify. Discover the symptoms that call for a visit to the doctor.

Exercise and diabetes

Exercise is crucial for managing diabetes, along with food and therapy. All forms of diabetes are consistent with this.

Maintaining an active lifestyle improves the way your cells respond to insulin and lowers blood sugar levels. You may also benefit from frequent exercise by:

Attain and maintain a healthy weight
Lower your risk of diabetes-related health issues
Increase mood
Sleep better

The overall recommendation is to strive for at least 150 minutes of moderate-intensity exercise per week if you have type 1 or type 2 diabetes. There aren't any specific workout recommendations for those with gestational diabetes at the moment. But to prevent overdoing it when pregnant, start carefully and gradually increase your exercise level over time.

Diabetes-friendly workouts consist of:

Walking
Cycling
Dancing
Swimming

Discuss safe methods to include exercise in your diabetes care strategy with your doctor. You may need to take extra measures, such as monitoring your blood sugar levels before and after working exercise and keeping hydrated.

Think about hiring a personal trainer or exercise physiologist who has knowledge of working with diabetics. They may assist you in creating a unique fitness schedule catered to your requirements.

Diagnosis of diabetes

Anyone who is at risk for developing diabetes or has symptoms should be tested. During the second or third trimester of pregnancy, women are often checked for gestational diabetes.

Doctors use these blood tests to identify prediabetes and diabetes:

Having fasted for eight hours, the fasting plasma glucose (FPG) test analyzes your blood sugar level.
An overview of your blood sugar levels over the last three months is given by the A1C test.

Diabetes avoidance

Because type 1 diabetes is an immune system disorder, it cannot be prevented. You also do not influence certain type 2 diabetes factors, such as your genes or age.

However, many more diabetes risk factors are controllable. The majority of diabetes preventive techniques include making small changes to your diet and exercise regimen.

Here are some steps you may take to put off developing type 2 diabetes if you have been diagnosed with prediabetes:

Get 150 minutes or more of cardiovascular activity each week by cycling or walking.

Eliminate refined carbs, saturated and trans fats from your diet.
Consume more whole grains, fruits, and veggies.
Consume lesser amounts.
If you are overweight or obese, try to shed 5% to 7% of your body weight.
There are more ways of avoiding diabetes than these. Learn more about the methods that might prevent this ongoing medical issue.

Takeaway

Some forms of diabetes, such as type 1, are brought on by external sources. Others, like type 2, may be avoided by improving dietary habits, increasing physical activity, and decreasing weight.

With your doctor, go through the dangers of diabetes. Have your blood sugar checked if you're at risk, and then manage your blood sugar according to your doctor's recommendations.

What are the types of diabetes?

Diabetes refers to a collection of diseases in which the body either cannot create enough or any insulin, cannot utilize the insulin that is produced correctly, or cannot do either of these things simultaneously.

The body is unable to transport sugar from the blood into your cells when any of these things take place. Blood sugar levels may rise as a result of this.

One of your primary energy sources is glucose, a kind of sugar present in your blood. Sugar builds up in your blood as a result of insulin deficiency or insulin resistance. Health issues may result from this.

There are three primary types of diabetes:

Type 1 diabetes
Type 2 diabetes
Gestational diabetes

Diabetes types

There are many varieties of diabetes:

Type 1:

Type 1 Diabetes is an autoimmune condition. The immune system targets and kills insulin-producing cells in the pancreas. Uncertainty surrounds the attack's origin. It is thought that type 1 diabetes is an autoimmune disorder. This implies that your immune system accidentally targets and kills the beta cells in your pancreas that are responsible for producing insulin. The harm is irreparable. The cause of the assaults remains unclear. Both hereditary and environmental factors may have a role. It is thought that lifestyle variables are not significant.

Type 2:

When your body gets resistant to insulin, type 2 diabetes develops and blood sugar levels rise. About 90% to 95%Trusted Source of persons with diabetes have type 2, making it the most prevalent kind. The first stage of type 2 diabetes is insulin resistance. This implies that since your body does not use insulin effectively, your pancreas produces more insulin until it is unable to meet the demand. The subsequent reduction in insulin synthesis results in elevated blood sugar.

Type 2 diabetes is not known to have a specific etiology. Potential contributing elements include:

Genetics and a sedentary way of life
Larger size or obesity
Other health and environmental variables might also have a role.

Gestational diabetes :

Gestational diabetes is excessive blood sugar when pregnant. This kind of diabetes is brought on by substances the placenta secretes that block insulin. Despite having a similar name to diabetes mellitus, the uncommon illness known as diabetes insipidus is unrelated. Your kidneys are removed from your body too much fluid in a separate ailment. Each kind of diabetes has specific symptoms, underlying conditions, and therapies. The pregnancy-related production of insulin-blocking substances results in gestational diabetes.

Pregnancy is the only time this form of diabetes occurs. People with previous prediabetes and a family history of diabetes are more likely to experience it.

Approximately half of women with gestational diabetes go on to acquire type 2 diabetes.

Type 1 diabetes symptoms may include:

Extreme thirst induced by hunger results in inadvertent weight loss
Frequent urination fatigue and blurred eyesight

It could also cause a shift in mood.

Type 2 diabetes symptoms may include:

Increased appetite
Heightened thirst
Increased urination, fatigue, and blurred vision
Taking a long time to cure sores
Moreover, it could lead to recurrent infections. This is because the body has a tougher time healing when glucose levels are high.

Pregnancy diabetes

The majority of women who acquire gestational diabetes show no symptoms. When doing a regular oral glucose tolerance test or blood sugar test, which is often done between the 24th and 28th week of pregnancy, medical professionals frequently find the issue.

A person with gestational diabetes may, in very rare circumstances, also feel increased thirst or urination.

In conclusion

Diabetes symptoms might be so subtle that they are first difficult to identify. Discover the symptoms that call for a visit to the doctor.

Diabetes causes

Each form of diabetes has a unique set of reasons.

Type 1 diabetes

Type 1 diabetes has an unknown specific etiology, according to doctors. The immune system wrongly targets and kills insulin-producing beta cells in the pancreas for some unknown cause. Some people may be affected by their genes. Additionally, a virus may trigger an immune system assault.

Type 2 diabetes

The cause of type 2 diabetes is a result of both hereditary and environmental factors. Your risk is further increased if you are overweight or obese. The effects of insulin on your blood sugar are resisted by your cells more when you are overweight, particularly in the abdomen.

Families are prone to this problem. Family members have genes that increase their risk of type 2 diabetes and obesity.

Pregnancy diabetes

Hormonal changes during pregnancy are the cause of gestational diabetes. The placenta secretes hormones that reduce the sensitivity of a pregnant person's cells to the effects of insulin. Pregnancy-related elevated blood sugar might result from this.

Gestational diabetes is more likely to develop in people who are overweight before becoming pregnant or who put on too much weight while pregnant.

Risk factors for diabetes

Your risk of diabetes is influenced by several things.

Type 1 diabetes

Type 1 diabetes is more common among children and teenagers, those who have a parent or sibling who has the illness, and people who have particular genes connected to the condition.

Type 2 diabetes

You are more likely to develop type 2 diabetes if you:

Age 45 or older
Overweight
Inactive
Have a parent or sibling with the illness
Had gestational diabetes, prediabetes, high blood pressure, high cholesterol, or high triglycerides, or have any of the following conditions:

Additionally, certain racial and ethnic groups are disproportionately affected by type 2 diabetes.

According to data from 2016, individuals of African American, Hispanic or Latino American, or Asian American heritage are more likely than white adults to be diagnosed with type 2 diabetes. Additionally, they are more likely to encounter worse treatment and greater self-management challenges.

Gestational diabetes

You are more likely to develop gestational diabetes if you:

Are obese

Are older than 25

Had gestational diabetes in a previous pregnancy

Have polycystic ovary syndrome (PCOS)

Have given birth to a child who weighed more than 9 pounds

Diabetes complications

Your body's organs and tissues are harmed by high blood sugar. Your risk of problems increases as your blood sugar level rises and as you live with it for a longer period of time.

Difficulties with diabetes

Your body's organs and tissues are harmed by high blood sugar. Your risk of problems increases as your blood sugar level rises and as you live with it for a longer period of time.

Diabetes-related complications include:

Stroke.
Heart attack, and heart disease
Neuropathy
Nephropathy
Retinopathy and reduced eyesight
Loss of hearing
Foot damage, including bacterial and fungal infections, non healing wounds, and infections and sores
Depression\dementia

Gestational Diabetes

Gestational diabetes that is not treated might result in issues for both the mother and the unborn child. Baby-related complications may take the following forms:

Early delivery
Higher-than-average birth weight, and a greater chance of developing type 2 diabetes later in life
Jaundice
Stillbirth

A woman who has gestational diabetes during pregnancy runs the risk of getting type 2 diabetes or high blood pressure (preeclampsia). You can also need a C-section, often known as a cesarean birth.

How widespread is diabetes?

In the United States, there are about 37.3 million persons with diabetes. Type 1 diabetes affects 5 to 10 percent of people, but type 2 affects 90 to 95 percent.

It is estimated that 84.1 million more persons have prediabetes. However, the majority of persons with prediabetes are unaware of their illness.

When your blood sugar is higher than it should be but not high enough to qualify as diabetes, you have prediabetes.

If you have a history of diabetes in your family, you are more likely to get the condition.

The following are additional type 2 diabetes risk factors:

Having a sedentary lifestyle
Being overweight or obese
Having experienced prediabetes or gestational diabetes

How are various forms of diabetes managed?

Whatever form of diabetes you have, managing it will need constant collaboration with your doctor.

Maintaining blood glucose levels within your desired range is the primary objective. Your desired range will be specified by your doctor. The type of diabetes, age, and presence of comorbidities all affect the targets.

Your blood sugar goals will be lower if you have gestational diabetes than if you have another form of diabetes.

Getting exercise is crucial for managing diabetes. Find out from your doctor how many minutes a week you should spend exercising aerobically. Nutrition is also crucial.

You must also keep an eye on your cholesterol and blood pressure.

Type 1 treatment:

Since pancreatic damage from type 1 diabetes is irreversible, all patients with the condition must take insulin to survive. Different insulin kinds are available, each with a unique onset, peak, and duration.

The skin-level injection of insulin occurs. Your doctor will demonstrate how to rotate injection sites and inject safely. A device worn outside of your body called an insulin pump, which may be set to release a precise dosage, is another option.

These days, you may get continuous blood glucose monitors that continuously check your blood sugar.

You must keep an eye on your blood sugar levels all day long. You may also need to take medicine to control your cholesterol, high blood pressure, or other issues, as appropriate.

Type 2 treatment

With proper nutrition and exercise, type 2 diabetes may be controlled and sometimes even reversed. To assist control blood sugar, it may also be treated using a range of drugs.

Metformin is generally the first-line drug (Glumetza, Glucophage, Fortamet, Riomet). This medication works by lowering the liver's ability to produce glucose. If metformin is ineffective, your doctor may recommend another drug.

You'll need to keep an eye on your blood sugar levels constantly. Additionally, you may need medicine to control your cholesterol and blood pressure.

Prevention

Type 1 diabetes has no recognized preventative measures.

Your risk of type 2 diabetes may be decreased if you:

Manage your weight
Concentrate on a nutrient-rich diet.
Engage in regular exercise.
Abstain from smoking
Have high triglycerides and low HDL cholesterol levels.

These behaviors may postpone or stop the establishment of type 2 diabetes if you already have prediabetes or gestational diabetes.

Outlook:

Type 1 diabetes does not have a treatment. Disease management must be ongoing. But with regular monitoring and commitment to the prescribed course of action, you may be able to prevent more severe disease-related consequences.

Type 2 diabetes is often effectively treated or even reversible if you work closely with your doctor and adopt a healthy lifestyle.

If you have gestational diabetes, it should go away after the birth of your child. You do, however, have a larger chance of getting type 2 diabetes in later life.

Chapter 2

- **What is diabetic neuropathy?**
- **Stress: How It Affects Diabetes and How to Decrease It**

All the Information You Need to Know About Diabetic Neuropathy

Diabetic neuropathy: what is it?

A critical and frequent consequence of both type 1 and type 2 diabetes is diabetic neuropathy. It is a kind of nerve injury brought on by persistently high blood sugar. The illness often takes years or even decades to fully manifest.

Consult your doctor if you have diabetes and have pain, tingling, numbness, or weakness in your hands or feet. These are peripheral neuropathy's first signs and symptoms. The risk generally arises when an ulcer forms on your foot and you are unable to feel pain.

If your peripheral neuropathy is severe or has persisted for a while, you might be more susceptible to wounds or infections. Amputation may be necessary for severe circumstances due to infection or poor wound healing.

Different kinds of diabetic neuropathy affect various body parts and result in a range of symptoms. It's crucial to constantly monitor your blood glucose levels if you have diabetes and to inform your doctor if you have any neuropathy symptoms.

What signs of diabetic neuropathy are there?

Neuropathy symptoms often come on gradually. The nerves in the foot are often the first to suffer from nerve injury. This may cause the sensation of "pins and needles" in your feet, which may be sometimes excruciating.

Depending on the locations impacted, symptoms change. The following are typical indicators and

Symptoms of the various forms of diabetic neuropathy:

The capacity for touch
Loss of touch
Trouble walking with balance
Numbness or discomfort in your hands or feet
Particularly at night, burning feeling in your feet
Wasting or weakening of the muscles
Bloating or fullness
Diarrhea or constipation
Dizziness when you stand up
Nausea
Indigestion, or vomiting
Excessive or reduced sweating
Bladder issues, including vaginal dryness and insufficient bladder emptying
Inability to recognize low blood sugar symptoms
Double vision
Erectile dysfunction
Higher heart rate

What variations of diabetic neuropathy are there?

Numerous forms of nerve injury are referred to as neuropathies. There are four basic forms of neuropathy in diabetics.

1: Peripheral neuropathy

Peripheral neuropathy is the most prevalent kind of neuropathy. Although it may also affect the arms or hands, peripheral neuropathy often affects the feet and legs. Different symptoms might range from moderate to severe. They consist of:

Numbness
High sensitivity to touch
Tingling or burning sensation
Lack of sensitivity to hot or cold temperatures
Acute discomfort or weak, cramping muscles
Lack of coordination or balance
Some people are more susceptible to their symptoms at night.

You may not feel an injury or discomfort on your foot if you have peripheral neuropathy. Diabetes patients often have impaired circulation, which makes healing wounds more challenging. Infection risk is increased by this mixture. In severe circumstances, an infection might result in amputation.

2: Autonomic neuropathy

Autonomic neuropathy is the second most common kind of neuropathy in diabetics.

Other bodily functions that you are unconscious of are controlled by the autonomic nervous system. It regulates a variety of muscles and organs, including your:

Cardiovascular system
Genitalia
Sweat glands
Sex organs
Digestive issues

Digestive system nerve injury may result in:

Constipation
Diarrhea
Problems swallowing.
Gastroparesis, in which the stomach empties into the small intestines too slowly.

Delays in digestion brought on by gastroparesis might become worse with time, resulting in frequent nausea and vomiting. Usually, you won't be able to complete a meal since you'll feel full too fast.

Blood glucose regulation is sometimes made more challenging by delayed digestion, with frequent swings between high and low values.

Additionally, individuals with autonomic neuropathy may not notice hypoglycemic signs like perspiration and heart palpitations. This may result in you being unaware that you have low blood sugar, which raises the possibility of a hypoglycemia emergency.

- **Bladder and sexual issues**

Sexual issues including the inability to have an orgasm, dry vagina, or erectile dysfunction may also be brought on by autonomic neuropathy. Bladder neuropathy may result in incontinence or make it challenging to empty your bladder.

- **Cardiovascular conditions**

Slower response times may result from damage to the nerves that regulate your heart rate and blood pressure. When you rise after laying down or sitting down, your blood pressure may drop, and you can feel faint or lightheaded. This can also happen when you exert yourself. An unusually rapid heart rate may also be brought on by autonomic neuropathy.

Some heart attack symptoms may be difficult to recognize if you have autonomic neuropathy. When your heart isn't receiving enough oxygen, you may not experience any chest discomfort. If you have autonomic neuropathy, you should be aware of additional heart attack warning symptoms, such as:

Profuse shortness of breath
Nausea
Discomfort in the arm, back, neck, jaw, or stomach.
Lightheadedness

- **Proximal neuropathy**

Proximal neuropathy, commonly known as diabetic amyotrophy, is an uncommon kind of neuropathy. This kind of neuropathy is more often seen in males and people over 50 with type 2 diabetes who have reasonably well-controlled blood sugar levels.

Frequently, the hips, buttocks, or thighs are affected. You could feel sudden, sometimes severe discomfort. Your legs' weakened muscles could make it challenging to stand up alone. One side of the body is often affected by diabetic amyotrophy.

Once symptoms start, they often become worse before slowly starting to get better. Fortunately, even without therapy, the majority of patients recover within a few years.

- **Focal neuropathy**

When a single nerve or set of nerves is damaged, the result is focal neuropathy, also known as mononeuropathy, which results in weakening in the afflicted region. You often experience this in your hand, head, body, or leg. It emerges out of nowhere and often hurts a lot.

Most focal neuropathies disappear after a few weeks or months, much like proximal neuropathy, and do not cause any long-term harm. Carpal tunnel syndrome is by far the most typical form.

About 25% of patients with diabetes have some level of nerve compression at the wrist, even though the majority do not have carpal tunnel syndrome symptoms.

The following are signs of focal neuropathy:

Inability to concentrate
Tingling
Discomfort in the fingers
Double vision and eye pain
Bell's palsy
Discomfort in specific locations, such as the big toe or the inside of the foot, the lower back, the pelvic area, the chest, or the stomach.

What is the root of diabetic neuropathy?

An extended duration of sustained elevated blood sugar levels leads to diabetic neuropathy. Nerve injury may also result from other sources, such as:

High cholesterol levels might lead to blood vessel damage.

Mechanical harm, such harm brought on by carpal tunnel syndrome

Lifestyle choices like drinking or smoking

Neuropathy may also result from low vitamin B-12 levels. Vitamin B-12 levels may be decreased by the popular diabetic drug metformin. You might request a quick blood test from your doctor to check for vitamin deficiencies.

Diagnosing diabetic neuropathy

A doctor will question you about your symptoms and medical history to start determining whether or not you have neuropathy. Additionally, you'll be physically examined. They will measure your heart rate, blood pressure, muscle tone, and degree of sensitivity to warmth and touch.

To determine how sensitive your feet are, your doctor could do a filament test. To do this, they'll evaluate your limbs for any loss of feeling using nylon fiber. You might measure your vibration threshold with a tuning fork. Your ankle reflexes may also be evaluated by your doctor.

The treatment for diabetic neuropathy

Diabetic neuropathy cannot be cured, however, it may be prevented from progressing as quickly. The greatest method to reduce the risk of developing diabetic neuropathy or limit its development is to maintain appropriate blood sugar levels. Additionally, it helps with certain symptoms.

A thorough treatment plan should also include regular exercise and quitting smoking. Before starting a new workout regimen, always with your doctor or healthcare team. Inquire with your physician about supplementary therapies or neuropathy supplements.

Treatment of pain

The discomfort brought on by diabetic neuropathy may be managed with medication. Discuss the available drugs with your doctor, as well as any possible adverse effects. It has been shown that a number of drugs may reduce symptoms.

Acupuncture is one alternative therapy that you may wish to take into account. Capsaicin has been discovered by certain studies to be beneficial. When combined with medicine, alternative treatments could provide more alleviation.

Managing difficulties

Your doctor may advise drugs, treatments, or lifestyle modifications depending on the kind of neuropathy you have to manage symptoms and prevent problems.

For instance, your doctor may advise you to eat smaller meals more often and restrict the amount of fiber and fat in your diet if your neuropathy is causing digestive issues.

Your doctor could recommend a lubricant if you suffer dryness in your vagina. They may recommend a medicine that may assist if you have erectile dysfunction.

Diabetes patients often have peripheral neuropathy, which may cause major foot problems and even amputation. If you have peripheral neuropathy, it's crucial to take extra care of your feet and to get medical attention right away if you become injured or uncomfortable.

Can diabetic neuropathy be avoided?

If you watch your blood glucose levels closely, you may often prevent developing diabetic neuropathy. Being consistent with:

Keeping an eye on your blood sugar levels
Controlling your nutrition

Taking prescribed medicines
Staying active

If you do get diabetic neuropathy, work closely with your doctor to minimize its growth according to their advice. You may lessen the harm done to your nerves and prevent problems by taking the appropriate care.

How Stress Affects Diabetes and How to Reduce Stress

Stress causes the body to produce hormones that may raise blood sugar levels. Diabetes patients may have negative effects from this, although they may be controlled.

Your body responds when you're under stress or feel threatened. The fight-or-flight reaction is what is meant by this.

Your body sends cortisol and adrenaline into the circulation during this reaction, and your breathing rate rises. If the body is unable to properly metabolize it, this may cause blood glucose levels to rise.

You might become psychologically and physically exhausted from ongoing stress caused by blood glucose issues that have persisted over time. This could make controlling your diabetes challenging.

What effects might stress have on your diabetes?

People respond to stress in various ways. Your body's reaction to stress might vary depending on the kind you encounter.

People with type 2 diabetes often notice a rise in their blood glucose levels when they are under emotional stress. People with type 1 diabetes could react differently. This indicates that their blood glucose levels may either rise or fall.

Your blood sugar might rise as a result of physical stress. This may occur as a result of an illness or accident. Both type 1 and type 2 diabetics may be impacted by this.

How can you tell whether your blood sugar levels are being impacted by mental stress?

You may be able to identify certain triggers by keeping note of extra details like the date and what you were doing when you were anxious.

Do you, for instance, usually feel stressed on Monday mornings? If so, you are aware of the specific actions you should take on Monday mornings to reduce stress and control your blood sugar.

By monitoring your stress and glucose levels, you can ascertain whether this is taking place for you.

Find out more about identifying the stress-related factors here.

You should measure your blood sugar levels after assessing your degree of stress. For the next several weeks, keep doing this. You may see a trend soon enough.

Your blood sugar is probably being adversely affected by your mental tension if you discover that it is consistently high.

What signs of stress are there?

You may not recognize stress's subtler side effects at first. Stress may have an influence on your physical health as well as your mental and emotional wellbeing. You may detect stress and manage it by recognizing the signs.

Among the physical signs of stress are:

Headaches
Muscular strain or discomfort
Widespread thoughts of disease while sleeping excessively or insufficiently
Fatigue

Additional symptoms of stress include:

Unmotivated
Irritable
Depressed
Restless
Anxious
Stressed individuals often exhibit behavior that may be uncharacteristic, such as:

Withdrawal from family and friends
Acting out of rage
Eating too much or too little
Drinking too much alcohol, and smoking

How to lessen your levels of stress

The pressures in your life may be reduced or limited. Here are some strategies you may use to control the consequences of various types of stress.

Regular exercise
Calming pursuits like yoga or tai chi.
Mindfulness exercises like meditation
Avoid well-known stressors, such tense social settings
Lessen your caffeine intake
Time with family and friends

How to manage stress caused by diabetes

Be assured that you are not alone if you are feeling anxious about your health. For solidarity and support, you may connect with individuals online or in your neighborhood.

Online forums for assistance

Online support groups may provide you with a strong network and practical advice to help you survive. For instance, the online resource Diabetic Connect aims to enhance your quality of life. It offers instructional films, recipes, and articles.

Localized support networks

Diabetes Sisters provides countrywide gatherings for female diabetics. It provides nationwide in-person gatherings.

Peer support groups are listed by the Defeat Diabetes Foundation in all 50 states and the District of Columbia. You may even browse the directory and add your own entry. Local offices of the American Diabetes Association that concentrate on community engagement and education are also available.

Therapy

Speaking about your stress with a professional could make you feel more at ease. A therapist can provide you coping skills that are specific to your circumstance and a secure setting in which to communicate. They could also give medical guidance that offline or online support groups are unable to.

What you can do right now

Despite the unique obstacles that diabetes might bring, it is possible to properly manage it and live a happy, healthy existence. You may include brief meditations or quick exercises into your everyday schedule. Find a support group that best fits your personality and lifestyle demands by researching support groups. Being a proactive person may help you de-stress.

Summary

Adrenaline and cortisol may be released into the blood as a result of both physical and mental stress. Blood glucose levels may increase as a result of these hormones.

Unexpected spikes in blood sugar may have a severe effect on a person's ability to control their diabetes and cause unpleasant symptoms. But being aware of stressors and using relaxation methods may help individuals deal with these situations.

Chapter 3

- **Healthy food, recipes and drinks when diagnosed with diabetes**
- **Low Carb Dinners for Type 1 Diabetes Made Easy**
- **Seven-Day Type 2 Diabetes Meal Plan**

Sorting out the best food varieties to eat when you have diabetes doesn't need to be intense.

To keep things straightforward, your fundamental objective ought to deal with your glucose levels.

It's additionally essential to eat food varieties that assist with forestalling diabetes inconveniences like coronary illness.

Your eating routine can play a significant part in forestalling and overseeing diabetes.

Here are the 16 best food varieties for individuals living with diabetes, both type 1 and type 2.

Best food varieties for individuals living with diabetes

1. Greasy fish

Salmon, sardines, herring, anchovies, and mackerel are extraordinary wellsprings of the omega-3 unsaturated fats DHA and EPA, which have significant advantages for heart wellbeing. Getting enough of these fats consistently is particularly significant for individuals with diabetes, who have an expanded gamble of coronary illness and stroke.

DHA and EPA safeguard the cells that line your veins, diminish markers of aggravation, and may assist with further developing how your supply routes capability.

Research demonstrates that individuals who eat greasy fish consistently have a lower hazard of intense coronary conditions, similar to cardiovascular failures, and are less inclined to kick the bucket from coronary illness. Concentrates on the show that eating greasy fish may likewise assist with controlling glucose.

A review including 68 grown-ups who had overweight or corpulence found that members who consumed greasy fish had critical enhancements in post-dinner glucose levels than members who consumed lean fish.

Fish is likewise an extraordinary wellspring of top-notch protein, which helps you feel full and balances out glucose levels.

In a nutshell

Greasy fish contain omega-3 fats that can assist with diminishing aggravation and other gamble variables of coronary illness and stroke. Furthermore, it's an extraordinary wellspring of protein, which is significant for overseeing glucose.

2. Salad greens

Verdant green vegetables are very nutritious and low in calories. They're additionally exceptionally low in edible carbs, or carbs consumed by the body, so they will not fundamentally influence glucose levels. Spinach, kale, and other mixed greens are great wellsprings of numerous nutrients and minerals, including L-ascorbic acid.

Some proof recommends that individuals with diabetes have lower L-ascorbic acid levels than individuals without diabetes, and they might have more noteworthy L-ascorbic acid prerequisites. L-ascorbic acid goes about as a powerful cell reinforcement and has mitigating characteristics.

Expanding dietary admission of L-ascorbic acid rich food varieties can assist individuals with diabetes to increase their serum L-ascorbic acid levels while diminishing aggravation and cell harm.

In a nutshell

Verdant green vegetables are plentiful in supplements like L-ascorbic acid as well as cancer prevention agents that safeguard your heart and eye wellbeing.

3. Avocados

Avocados have under 1 gram of sugar, scarcely any starches, a high fiber content, and solid fats, so you don't need to stress over them raising your glucose levels.

Avocado utilization is additionally connected with further developed generally speaking eating routine quality and fundamentally lower body weight and weight record (BMI).

This makes avocados an optimal nibble for individuals with diabetes, particularly since corpulence expands the possibilities of creating diabetes.

Avocados might have properties well defined for forestalling diabetes.

A recent report in mice found that avocatin B (AvoB), a fat particle tracked down just in avocados, represses fragmented oxidation in skeletal muscle and the pancreas, which diminishes insulin obstruction.

More examination is required in people to lay out the association between avocados and diabetes counteraction.

In a nutshell

Avocados have under 1 gram of sugar and are related with further developed generally speaking eating routine quality. Avocados may likewise have properties well defined for diabetes counteraction.

4. Eggs

Customary egg utilization might diminish your coronary illness risk in more ways than one.

Eggs might diminish aggravation, further develop insulin responsiveness, increment your HDL (great) cholesterol levels, and change the size and state of your LDL (terrible) cholesterol.

A recent report found that eating a high-fat, low-carb breakfast of eggs could assist individuals with diabetes oversee glucose levels for the day.

More established research has connected egg utilization with coronary illness in individuals with diabetes.

In any case, a later survey of controlled examinations found that eating 6 to 12 eggs each week as a component of a nutritious eating routine didn't increase coronary illness risk factors in individuals with diabetes.

Additionally, some exploration recommends that eating eggs might diminish the gamble of stroke.

In a nutshell

Eggs might further develop risk factors for coronary illness, advance great glucose in the executives, safeguard eye wellbeing, and keep you feeling full.

5. Chia seeds

Chia seeds are magnificent nourishment for individuals with diabetes. They're very high in fiber, yet low in absorbable carbs.

11 of the 12 grams of carbs in a 28-gram (1-ounce) serving of chia seeds are fiber, which doesn't raise glucose. The gooey fiber in chia seeds can bring down your glucose levels by

dialing back the rate at which food travels through your stomach and is assimilated.

Chia seeds might assist you with accomplishing a moderate weight since fiber diminishes yearning and encourages you. Chia seeds may likewise help keep up with glycemic executives in individuals with diabetes.

A review including 77 grown-ups with overweight or corpulence and a determination of type 2 diabetes found that eating chia seeds upholds weight reduction and keeps up with great glycemic control.

Furthermore, chia seeds have been displayed to assist with diminishing circulatory strain and provocative markers.

In a nutshell

Chia seeds contain high measures of fiber, which might assist you with getting in shape. They additionally assist with keeping up with blood glucose levels.

6. Beans

Beans are reasonable, nutritious, and very sound. Beans are a sort of vegetable plentiful in B nutrients, valuable minerals (calcium, potassium, and magnesium), and fiber. They likewise have an exceptionally low glycemic record, which is significant for overseeing diabetes. Beans may likewise assist with forestalling diabetes.

In a review including more than 3,000 members at high risk of cardiovascular sickness, the people who had higher utilization of vegetables had a diminished possibility of creating type 2 diabetes.

In a nutshell

Beans are modest, nutritious, and have a low glycemic record, making them a solid choice for individuals with diabetes.

7. Greek yogurt

A drawn-out study including well-being information from more than 100,000 members observed that a day-to-day serving of yogurt was connected to an 18 percent lower chance of creating type 2 diabetes.

It might likewise assist you with getting in shape, on the off chance that that is an individual objective.

Concentrating on yogurt and other dairy food varieties might prompt weight reduction and further develop body organization in individuals with type 2 diabetes.

The elevated degrees of calcium, protein and an extraordinary sort of fat called formed linoleic corrosive (CLA) found in yogurt might assist with keeping you full for longer.

Additionally, Greek yogurt contains just 6-8 grams of carbs per serving, which is lower than traditional yogurt.

It's additionally higher in protein, which might advance weight reduction by diminishing craving and along these lines diminishing calorie consumption.

In a nutshell

Yogurt might advance sound glucose levels, decrease risk factors for coronary illness, and help with weight the executives.

8. Nuts

Nuts are scrumptious and nutritious. Most sorts of nuts contain fiber and are low in net carbs, albeit some have more than others.

Research on a wide range of nuts has shown that customary utilization might diminish irritation and lower glucose, HbA1c (a marker for long haul glucose in the executives), and LDL (terrible) cholesterol levels.

Nuts may likewise assist individuals with diabetes in further developing their heart well-being.

A recent report including over 16,000 members with type 2 diabetes found that eating tree nuts — like pecans, almonds, hazelnuts, and pistachios — brought down their gamble of coronary illness and passing. Research additionally demonstrates that nuts can further develop blood glucose levels. A review of individuals with type 2 diabetes found that eating pecan oil day to day superior blood glucose levels.

This finding is significant because individuals with type 2 diabetes frequently have raised degrees of insulin, which are connected to corpulence.

In a nutshell

Nuts are a sound expansion to a reasonable eating routine. They're high in fiber and can assist with diminishing glucose and LDL (terrible) cholesterol levels.

9. Broccoli

Broccoli is one of the most nutritious vegetables around. A half cup of cooked broccoli contains just 27 calories and 3 grams of edible carbs, alongside significant supplements like L-ascorbic acid and magnesium. Broccoli may likewise assist with dealing with your glucose levels.

One investigation discovered that consuming broccoli sprouts prompted a decrease in blood glucose in individuals with diabetes.

This decrease in blood glucose levels is reasonable due to sulforaphane, a substance in cruciferous vegetables like broccoli and fledglings.

In a nutshell

Broccoli is a low-calorie, low-carb food with high supplement esteem. It's stacked with solid plant intensities that might help safeguard against different infections.

10. Extra-virgin olive oil

Extra-virgin olive oil contains oleic corrosive, a kind of monounsaturated fat that might improve glycemic the executives, diminish fasting and post-dinner fatty substance levels, and has cell reinforcement properties.

This is significant because individuals with diabetes will generally experience difficulty overseeing glucose levels and have high fatty substance levels.

Oleic corrosive may likewise invigorate the completion chemical GLP-1.

In an enormous examination of 32 investigations taking a gander at various kinds of fat, olive oil was the only one displayed to decrease coronary illness risk.

Olive oil additionally contains cancer prevention agents called polyphenols.

Polyphenols diminish aggravation, safeguard the cells covering your veins, hold oxidation back from harming your LDL (terrible) cholesterol, and abate circulatory strain.

Extra-virgin olive oil is crude, so it holds cancer prevention agents and different properties that work everything out.

Make certain to pick extra-virgin olive oil from a respectable source, since numerous olive oils are blended in with less expensive oils like corn and soy.

In a nutshell

Extra-virgin olive oil contains sound oleic corrosiveness. It has benefits for circulatory strain and heart wellbeing.

11. Flaxseeds

Otherwise called normal flax or linseeds, flaxseeds have a highly satisfied heart-solid omega-3 fats, fiber, and other one-of-a-kind plant compounds.

A piece of their insoluble fiber is lignans, which might assist with diminishing coronary illness risk and further develop glucose in the executives.

A survey breaking down 25 randomized clinical preliminaries tracked down a critical relationship between entire flaxseed supplementation and a decrease in blood glucose (20).

Flaxseeds may likewise assist with bringing down circulatory strain.

A recent report including members with prediabetes found that a day-to-day admission of flaxseed powder brought down circulatory strain — however it didn't improve glycemic executives or insulin obstruction. More exploration is expected to research how flaxseed can help forestall or oversee diabetes. Be that as it may, generally speaking, flaxseed is advantageous for your heart and stomach wellbeing.

Additionally, flaxseeds are exceptionally high in gooey fiber, which further develops stomach wellbeing, insulin responsiveness, and sensations of completion.

In a nutshell

Flaxseeds might assist with diminishing aggravation, lower coronary illness risk, decline glucose levels, and further develop insulin responsiveness.

12. Apple juice vinegar and vinegar

Apple juice vinegar and plain vinegar have numerous medical advantages. Even though it's produced using apples, the sugar in the organic product is matured into acidic corrosive. The subsequent item contains under 1 gram of carbs per tablespoon.

As indicated by a meta-investigation of six examinations, incorporating 317 individuals with type 2 diabetes, vinegar helpfully affects fasting glucose levels and HbA1c.

Apple juice vinegar might have numerous other invigorating properties, including antimicrobial and cancer prevention agent impacts. Be that as it may, more investigations are expected to affirm its medical advantages.

To integrate apple juice vinegar into your eating routine, start with 4 teaspoons blended in a glass of water every day before dinner. Note that you might need to put 1 teaspoon for every glass of water so the taste isn't a serious area of strength for as. Increment to a limit of 4 tablespoons each day.

In a nutshell

Apple juice vinegar might assist with further developing fasting glucose levels, however, more examination is expected to affirm its medical advantages.

13. Strawberries

Strawberries are high in cancer prevention agents known as anthocyanins, which give them their red tone. They additionally contain polyphenols, which are advantageous plant compounds with cancer prevention agent properties. A recent report tracked down that a 6-week utilization of polyphenols from strawberries and cranberries further developed insulin responsiveness in grown-ups with overweight and corpulence who didn't have diabetes.

This is significant because low insulin responsiveness can cause glucose levels to turn out to be excessively high.

A 1-cup serving of strawberries contains around 53.1 calories and 12.7 grams of carbs, three of which are fiber.

This serving likewise gives over 100 percent of the reference day-to-day admission (RDI) for L-ascorbic acid, which gives extra mitigating advantages to heart wellbeing.

In a nutshell

Strawberries are low-sugar organic products that have solid mitigating properties and may assist with further developing insulin obstruction.

14. Garlic

For its minuscule size and low carbohydrate content, garlic is extraordinarily nutritious.

One clove (3 grams) of crude garlic, which is approximately 4 calories, contains.

Manganese: 2% of the day-to-day esteem (DV)
Vitamin B6: 2% of the DV
L-ascorbic acid: 1% of the DV
Selenium: 1% of the DV
Fiber: 0.06 grams

Research demonstrates that garlic adds to further developed blood glucose executives and can assist with controlling cholesterol.

Albeit many investigations that decide garlic is a demonstrated sound choice for individuals living with diabetes incorporate unusual dietary measures of garlic, the meta-examination referred to above just included servings from 0.05-1.5 grams. For setting, one clove of garlic is around 3 grams. Research additionally demonstrates that garlic can assist with diminishing circulatory strain and control cholesterol levels.

In a nutshell

Garlic assists lower blood sugar, aggravation, LDL cholesterol, and circulatory strain in individuals with diabetes.

15. Squash

Squash, which has numerous assortments, is one of the best vegetables around. The thick, filling food is genuinely low in calories and has a low glycemic record. Winter assortments have a hard shell and incorporate oak seed, pumpkin, and butternut. Summer squash has a delicate strip that can be eaten. The most widely recognized types are zucchini and Italian squash. Like most vegetables, squash contains advantageous cancer prevention agents. Squash likewise has less sugar than yams, making it an extraordinary other option.

Research shows that pumpkin polysaccharides, which are additionally tracked down in squash, further developed insulin resistance and diminished degrees of serum glucose in rodents.

Although there's a tiny examination of people, a little report found that squash diminished high blood glucose levels rapidly and successfully in individuals with diabetes who were fundamentally sick. More investigations with people are expected to affirm the medical advantages of squash.

Be that as it may, the medical advantages of squash make it an extraordinary expansion to any dinner.

In a nutshell

Summer and winter squash contain advantageous cancer prevention agents and may assist with bringing down glucose.

16. Shirataki noodles

Shirataki noodles are magnificent for diabetes and weight executives. These noodles are high in the fiber glucomannan, which is extricated from konjac root. This plant is filled in Japan and handled into the state of noodles or rice known as shirataki.

Glucomannan is a kind of thick fiber, which helps you feel full and fulfilled. Additionally, it's been displayed to decrease glucose levels in the wake of eating and further develop coronary illness risk factors in individuals with diabetes and metabolic condition.

In one review, glucomannan fundamentally diminished degrees of fasting blood glucose, serum insulin, and cholesterol in rodents with diabetes.

A 3.5-ounce (100-gram) serving of shirataki noodles likewise contains only 3 grams of edible carbs and only 10 calories for every serving.

Notwithstanding, these noodles are ordinarily bundled with a fluid that has an off-putting scent, and you want to flush them a very long time before use. Then, at that point, to guarantee a noodle-like surface, cook the noodles for a few minutes in a skillet over high intensity without added fat.

In a nutshell

The glucomannan in shirataki noodles advances sensations of completion and can further develop glucose executives and cholesterol levels.

Food varieties to keep away from

Similarly as significant as sorting out which food varieties you ought to remember for an eating routine for diabetes is understanding which food varieties you ought to restrict.

This is because numerous food varieties and beverages are high in carbs and added sugar, which can cause glucose levels to spike.

Different food varieties could adversely influence heart wellbeing or add to weight gain.

The following are a couple of food varieties that you ought to restrict or stay away from on the off chance that you have diabetes.

1. Refined grains

Refined grains like white bread, pasta, and rice are high in carbs but low in fiber, which can increment glucose levels more rapidly than their entire grain partners.

As indicated by one examination survey, entire grain rice was fundamentally more successful at balancing out glucose levels in the wake of eating than white rice.

2. Sugar-improved refreshments

In addition to the fact that sugar is improved, refreshments like pop, sweet tea, and caffeinated drinks lack significant supplements, however, they additionally contain a concentrated measure of sugar in each serving, which can cause glucose levels to spike.

3. Broiled food varieties

Broiled food varieties have a great deal of trans fat, a kind of fat that has been connected to a higher gamble of coronary illness. Additionally, broiled food varieties like potato chips, french fries, and mozzarella sticks are additionally ordinarily high in calories, which could add to weight gain.

4. Liquor

Individuals with diabetes are for the most part encouraged to restrict their liquor consumption. This is because liquor can expand the gamble of low glucose, particularly whenever consumed while starving.

5. Breakfast cereal

Most assortments of breakfast cereal are exceptionally high in added sugar. A few brands pack as much sugar into a solitary filling in as certain pastries.

While looking for cereal, make certain to check the nourishment name cautiously and select an assortment that is low in sugar. On the other hand, settle on cereal and improve it normally with a touch of a new natural product.

6. Candy

Candy contains a high measure of sugar in each serving. It ordinarily has a high glycemic record, meaning it's probably going to cause spikes and crashes in glucose levels after you eat.

7. Handled meats

Handled meats like bacon, sausages, salami, and cold cuts are high in sodium, additives, and other destructive mixtures. Moreover, handled meats have been related to a higher gamble of coronary illness.

8. Natural product juice

Albeit 100 percent natural product juice can be delighted in every once in a while with some restraint, it's ideal to adhere to the entire natural product whenever the situation allows on the off chance that you have diabetes.

This is because organic product juice contains all the carbs and sugar tracked down in new natural products, however, it's deficient with regards to the fiber expected to assist with balancing out glucose levels.

Making an arrangement
There are a few methodologies you can use to design a solid, balanced diet for diabetes.

- **Plate technique**

The plate technique is a straightforward and successful method for supporting solid glucose levels without following or estimating your food. It expects you to change your segments of specific nutritional categories on your plate to make a healthfully adjusted dinner.

To get everything rolling, essentially fill around 50% of your plate with non-boring vegetables, like mixed greens, broccoli, squash, or cauliflower.

One-fourth of your plate ought to comprise proteins, similar to chicken, turkey, eggs, fish, tofu, and lean cuts of hamburger or pork.

The leftover quarter of the plate ought to contain a decent wellspring of sugars, including entire grains, vegetables, boring vegetables, natural products, or dairy items.

At long last, make certain to coordinate your dinner with a low-calorie refreshment to assist you with remaining hydrated, like water, unsweetened tea, dark espresso, or club pop.

- **Glycemic record**

The glycemic record can be a successful instrument for keeping up with glucose levels. It's utilized to quantify how much certain food varieties increment glucose levels and classifies them as high, low, or medium GI food in light of their glycemic record.

On the off chance that you utilize this technique, stick to food varieties with a low or medium glycemic record whenever the situation allows, and limit your admission of food varieties that have a high glycemic file.

You can track down more data about the glycemic record and how to utilize it to further develop glucose control in this article.

- **Carb counting**

Carb counting is a well-known technique used to oversee glucose levels by observing how much starches you consume for the day.

It includes following the grams of carbs in the food varieties you eat. Now and again, you may likewise have to change your measurements of insulin in light of how much carbs you consume.

The number of carbs you ought to eat for every dinner and tidbit can fluctuate a considerable amount contingent upon factors like your age, size, and movement level.

In this manner, an enrolled dietitian or specialist can assist you with making a modified arrangement for carb counting in light of your requirements.

Test menu

Eating sound with diabetes doesn't need to be troublesome or tedious.

Here is a 1-day test menu with some simple dinner thoughts to assist with kicking you off:

Breakfast: omelet with broccoli, mushrooms, and peppers
Morning nibble: a modest bunch of almonds
Lunch: a barbecued chicken serving of mixed greens with spinach, tomatoes, avocado, onions, cucumber, and balsamic vinaigrette
Evening nibble: Greek yogurt with cut strawberries and pecans
Supper: prepared salmon with spice quinoa and asparagus
Evening nibble: cut veggies and hummus

Important point

At the point when diabetes isn't all around made due, it expands your gamble of a few serious illnesses.

In any case, eating food varieties that assist with keeping glucose, insulin, and aggravation under tight restraints can emphatically decrease your gamble of entanglements.

Simply recollect, albeit these food varieties might assist with overseeing glucose, the main calculated sound glucose the executives are following a, generally speaking, nutritious, adjusted diet.

Low Carb Dinners for Type 1 Diabetes Made Easy

Cooking a sound, low carb supper can feel overpowering and monotonous toward the finish of a drawn out day, particularly on the off chance that you're not set up with simple fixings and a recognizable, low support cooking technique.

There are a ton of motivations to legitimize snatching takeout coming back from work, however cooking your own low carb supper made with entire food varieties can be exceptionally simple — also scrumptious.

I love preparing my own dinners, however, I despise going through my night on excessively convoluted recipes requiring a large number of fixings and lots of time.

All things being equal, I keep it straightforward, quick and brimming with different flavors. This is a shelter for my glucose executives and generally speaking well-being with type 1 diabetes (T1D).

We should investigate this simple method for cooking different solid suppers rapidly and with insignificant prep work or extravagant cooking abilities.

What number of carbs would it be a good idea for you to eat?
This is a significant spot to begin, as well as a sensitive subject for some. By the day's end, all that ultimately matters feels maintainable and suitable for you.

For the typical American, eating under 100 grams of starches each day is a sensational low carb exertion. For individuals with T1D, it's become more mind-boggling. The dependable guidelines are presently generally as adheres to:

Moderate, lower carb: under 100 grams of net starches each day

Low carb: under 50 grams of net starches each day

Ketogenic/Bernstein diet: under 20 grams of starch each day

Note that the expression "net starches" alludes to taking away dietary fiber from the complete carb amount to decide the carbs that will influence glucose.

For this article, we're centered around accomplishing lower or low carb eating by keeping away from boring vegetables and grains at supper, yet at the same time some of the time including some "higher carb" entire food vegetables, similar to carrots.

By and by, I've followed severe low carb and lower carb consumption fewer calories all through my 21 years of living with T1D. I've come to finish up a couple of individual convictions about what a solid eating routine with T1D resembles me:

Eat for the most part genuine food.

The end.
With or without mockery, my main nourishment prerequisite today is that 80 to 90 percent of my eating regimen (three out of four dinners) consistently comprises entire, genuine food fixings.

I eat natural products day to day. I eat dessert practically day to day. I eat vegetables (counting the starchier ones like corn and peas) three dinners every day. I save my more handled or boring starch decisions for dessert guilty pleasures.

On the off chance that it's a genuine food thing and I can sort out how much insulin I really want to cover it in the wake of eating on more than one occasion, then, at that point, it's great for me.

Eat genuine food. It's just straightforward. Strawberries aren't Satan since I really want to take insulin for them.

The way to deal with preparing low carb suppers centers around genuine fixings while staying away from the starchiest plants like potatoes, sweet potatoes, and grains.

A speedy and simple low carb supper approach
Two things make this piece of my eating regimen so extraordinarily simple:

Cook protein (anything from steak to tofu) in an air fryer.
Cook vegetables in steam and sauté technique that requires no additional water (which causes veggies to feel and possess a flavor like mush), yet just requires a teaspoon of oil.
I seriously hate fastidious recipes. This way to deal with cooking sound, entire food suppers is adaptable and fundamental.

It implies you can trade in any sort of vegetables and any kind of meat, changing simply the specific temperature or minutes without changing the strategies and generally speaking time it takes to finish.

We should investigate.

Why you ought to purchase an air fryer
As I would like to think, you really want an air fryer. And negative, it's not only for making french fries.

An air fryer is a tremendous piece of my "cook low carb suppers rapidly" methodology — particularly for cooking meat. Here's the reason:

It warms up such a great deal quicker than a broiler.
It figures out how to keep meat succulent while still giving it an "off the barbecue" flavor.
It's incredibly simple to clean.
You can get a respectable one for about $60 to $80.
It cooks the meat quickly.
No flipping or blending fundamentals.
You can likewise cook vegetables in it (old fashioned corn turns out awesome).

I genuinely utilize my air fryer a few times each day. I additionally never had trouble "preheating" it; that rarely makes a difference.

Instances of things I cook in my air fryer

Chicken. It for the most part requires preheating the broiler and afterward baking for 25 to 30 minutes. In an air fryer, the chicken should be possible in 12 to 20 minutes relying upon the size of the meat.
Breakfast frankfurter. I use it to cook these in the first part of the day while never stressing over it consuming on one side. Just "set it and fail to remember it." Seriously. Four minutes at 400°F (204°C) in the air fryer and it's finished. Functions admirably with my little girl's sausages, as well. So natural.
Steaks. I cook steaks in under 8 minutes. They come out completely like clockwork. No flipping.
Hard-bubbled eggs. You don't have to lounge around and trust that water will bubble. Just lay a couple of eggs in the air fryer container and set

it to 250°F (121°C) for 16 minutes or 300°F (149°C) for 12 minutes.
Tofu. Channel the water from the tofu compartment. Cut the tofu into solid shapes. Lay them scattered in the air fryer, set for 375°F (190.5°C) degrees for 15 to 20 minutes, and VOILA! The most mouth-watering tofu you'll at any point meet in your life.
Also natively constructed meatballs, crunchy "broiled" chicken, wings, drumsticks, burgers, diced-up chicken frankfurter, Italian hotdog, veggie burgers… you can cook anything. (But bacon — what a wreck!)

You can continuously open the air fryer and keep an eye on your food during the cooking system. On the off chance that it's not finished, simply close it back up and it cooks.

I genuinely don't cook meat in the broiler any longer except if I'm making a tremendous cluster of meatballs or a Thanksgiving turkey. I utilize my air fryer each day, on different occasions a day.

Figuring out how to steam and sauté: It's simple This technique for cooking vegetables is a blend of what's the big deal about steaming (it mellow vegetables without added fat) and sautéing (it gives them a crisper touch and preferable flavor over steaming).

In the first place, keep a decent supply of vegetables in your refrigerator that doesn't spoil rapidly. This implies you can purchase a lot of these veggies on Sunday and use them in dinners all week long. I keep a decent stockpile of these vegetables in my refrigerator every week:

Celery
Onion
Bean grows (an extraordinary substitution for pasta)
Broccoli (frozen pack functions admirably as well)
Carrots (purchase the pack of pre-sliced to save time on cleaving)
Zucchini

Summer squash
Green cabbage (higher in carbs than lettuce)
Purple cabbage (higher in carbs than lettuce)
scallions
Peas (frozen sack)

Then, at that point, pick three of these vegetables (in addition to an onion or scallion for flavor) and spot them in an enormous container that accompanies a tight cover, and follow these means:

Sprinkle 1 or 2 tsp. oil (olive, coconut, avocado, and so forth) on the veggies. Throw or mix rapidly to guarantee the oil is spread across the container piece.
Cover and turn the intensity to medium-high (or #7 on the burner dial).
Mix vegetables for the following 5 minutes, then, at that point, cover once more. (Water from the vegetables will act as a steaming source while the cover is on.)
After 5 to 8 minutes, when you can penetrate the vegetables with a fork, eliminate the cover and

mix consistently. This will sauté the vegetables, giving them a crispier appearance and flavor.
Sauté for an additional 5 minutes, roughly.
Switch off the intensity.
Add your favored salt and preparing blend (you can utilize a premixed mix from the store or keep it straightforward with salt and pepper) or your number one low carb dressing or sauce.
Fill around 50% of your plate with vegetables and add your protein. So natural!

Note: You can utilize CalorieKing to get a good guess of the carb included in your dinner. The vast majority of these blends will amount to less than 20 grams of net starches. (Likewise, an update that green and purple cabbage contain surprisingly starches.)

A couple of tips on utilizing spices and flavors
Salt isn't the adversary. Assuming your eating regimen comprises for the most part genuine food that you set yourself up at home, the main sodium in your eating regimen will to a great extent be what you put in it.

Notwithstanding, remember that on the off chance that you're utilizing different fun spices and flavors on the vegetables, you should keep the meat prepared more straightforward, or the other way around.

One more basic detail to consider — on the off chance that your eating regimen has recently been loaded up with a ton of vigorously handled and bundled things — is to give your taste buds time to adjust to the flavor of entire food varieties.

For instance, you don't have to add a lot of teriyaki sauce to broccoli for it to taste great. Attempt to let your taste buds reconstruct their appreciation for the unadulterated taste of entire food varieties.

Flavor tips for vegetables

Utilizing a flavor-pressed Himalayan pink salt in addition to different spices and flavors implies your taste buds can reconnect with the genuine kinds of vegetables as opposed to weighty fixings.

On the off chance that you're new to flavors, I suggest beginning with a portion of the premixed flavors in the baking passageway of your supermarket. Some of them might contain a smidgen of sugar, however, the sum that really winds up on your plate will be insignificant.

The following are a couple of simple combos to kick you off:

Salt + paprika + celery salt
Salt + thyme + rosemary
Garlic salt + Italian spice mix
Salt + Parmesan cheddar + celery salt
Salt + Parmesan cheddar + paprika
Flavor tips for meat
I should admit I'm really fixated on A.1. Steak Sauce, which is fundamentally improved and enhanced by raisins. A sprinkle of delightful Himalayan pink salt goes quite far as well.

Here are simple methods for flavoring meat:

Dry rubs. These are fundamentally only a flavoring mix scoured or moved onto meat before cooking.

Low sugar toppings. There are so many on the racks today that you can brush onto meat previously and during cooking.

Make your own. Use spices and flavors in addition to allulose for improving to make your own low-carb preparing mixes.

Olive oil and salt. Brush and sprinkle on meat before cooking.

Remember there are various ways you can apply flavor contingent upon your inclination. With chicken drums or thighs, for instance, you can place the meat into a bowl and delicately press or roll the meat in the bowl before setting it in the air fryer.

For meat that is cut or cubed before cooking, you can throw the meat bits while preparing in a bowl, or hold on until they're cooked and plated to sprinkle and prepare on top.

Some extraordinary low carb suppers to attempt Presently we should sort out a couple of my number one dinners utilizing the air fryer and steam/sauté techniques.

You'll ordinarily get the meat rolling first since that part takes the longest. While the meat is cooking, you can cleave and cook your veggies. I'm not determining amounts here, because the thought is that you can change as per your requirements. You don't have to break out the estimating cups and spoons to make simple, scrumptious veggie and meat dishes.

Italian Night

Ingredients

Italian frankfurter (pick turkey-based adaptations for lower fat choices)
Bean sprouts

Cut onion
Cut carrots
Parmesan cheddar
Salt
Garlic salt

Headings

Place Italian frankfurter in the air fryer.

Cook for 15 minutes at 350°F (176.6°C). Check to affirm it's cooked before serving by cutting one frankfurter open.

While the meat is cooking, cook veggies per steam/sauté headings above.

Whenever everything is cooked, add Parmesan cheddar, salt, and garlic salt to the vegetables.

Cut the frankfurters, then, at that point, plate, serve, and appreciate.

What likewise coordinates well with this dish is a number one of mine, this lower-carb edamame pasta.

Chicken Thighs and Zucchini Medley.

Ingredients

Chicken thighs
Caribbean Jerk mix
Cut onion
Cut zucchini
Cut carrots

Headings

Cover one side of every chicken thigh with Caribbean Jerk mix.
Place chicken thighs in the air fryer for 20 minutes at 375°F (190.5°C).
Add veggies to a griddle, and cover with top.
Cook per steam/sauté headings above.
Plate, serve, and appreciate.

Chicken Apple Sausage and Bean Sprout Medley

Ingredients

Aidells Chicken and Apple Sausage
cut onion
sack of bean sprouts
slashed celery

Himalayan pink salt
Parmesan cheddar
Bearings
Cut the frankfurters into reduced-down pieces.
Place in the air fryer and cook for 15 minutes at 350°F (176.6°C).
Place the veggies into a griddle.
Cook per steam/sauté headings above.
Add Himalayan pink salt and Parmesan cheddar to the veggies.
Plate, serve, and appreciate.

Steak, Onions, Sprouts, and Yellow Squash

Ingredients
steaks
slashed onion
slashed yellow squash
pack of bean sprouts
1-2 tsp. olive oil
Himalayan pink salt

Headings

Place steaks in the air fryer for 15 to 20 minutes (contingent upon how well you need them cooked) at 375°F (190.5°C).
Cleave the onion and yellow squash.
Add onion, squash, and sack of bean sprouts into a griddle with olive oil.
Cover with top and cook per stem/sauté bearings above.
Add Himalayan pink salt to the veggies and steak.
Plate, serve, and appreciate.

Low Carb 'Broiled' Chicken

Ingredients
chicken thighs or chicken fingers
low carb flour (chickpea, almond, or coconut)
1-2 whisked eggs
low carb breadcrumbs
your number one cleaved veggie combo
Headings
Cut up chicken thighs or tenders into finger-food pieces.

Put chicken pieces into an enormous zip-close sack.
Add 1/2 cup low-carb flour to the sack and shake until chicken is covered.
Add 1 whisked egg to the sack (add another egg if fundamental) and shake until chicken is covered.
Add low carb breadcrumbs to the sack and shake until chicken is covered.
Dump out of sight fryer containers.
Cook at 350-375°F (176.6-190.5°C) for 15-20 minutes.
Steam/sauté your veggies utilizing the bearings above while the chicken cooks.
Partake in the chicken with your number one plunge of decision.
Genuinely, cooking your own low carb suppers isn't unreasonably confusing, and it unquestionably doesn't need to take time-consuming.

Be that as it may, you do have to keep a decent inventory of veggies in the refrigerator or cooler, and stock a pleasant assortment of flavors, spices, flavors, and lower carb fixings to make the additional flavor.

It's an educational experience. Allow yourself to analyze. Disregard the Martha Stewart rulebook of recipes, and show restraint.

Truly, everything unquestionably revolves around essentially blending veggies in with protein sources and adding some scrumptious flavor!

Seven-Day Type 2 Diabetes Meal Plan

- **Day 1**

Eating a diabetes-accommodating eating routine can assist with monitoring your glucose levels. However, it very well may be hard to adhere to a customary feast plan — except if you have an arrangement set up.

Look at these 21 delightful, diabetes-accommodating recipes to use for breakfast, lunch, and supper. Make sure to remain inside your carb remittance by noticing the carb content and serving size of the recipes. Likewise, make certain to offset your dinners with lean protein and solid plant fats.

Breakfast: Cream Cheese-Stuffed French Toast

This might sound excessively wanton for breakfast, yet matched with fried egg whites, it can squeeze into a diabetes-accommodating dinner plan. Entire grain toast will assist with guaranteeing you get your everyday fiber as well.

Lunch: Salmon Salad with White Beans

Salmon is one of the most mind-blowing wellsprings of omega-3 unsaturated fats and is likewise a delightful clincher to business day salad.

Supper: Cuban-Marinated Sirloin Kabobs with Grilled Asparagus

Zest things up with this delightful stick. Dried spices and flavors are an extraordinary method for sneaking up all of a sudden of flavor without adding pointless calories and fat.

- **Day 2**

Breakfast: Apple Pie Oatmeal with Greek Yogurt

Who couldn't really care for a cut of pie for breakfast? This cereal will leave your kitchen possessing an aroma like the kind of fall, and your stomach cheerful and fulfilled. Add some additional plain Greek yogurt on top for more protein.

Lunch: Turkey-Cranberry Wraps

Turkey and cranberry sauce aren't only for Thanksgiving! This is a simple in-and-out lunch that even your children will appreciate.

Note: This recipe may not be fitting for all individuals with type 2 diabetes, since it contains 60 grams of carbs per serving. You can change how much cranberry sauce to bring down the carb count.

Supper: Cilantro-Lime Tilapia with Spinach and Tomatoes

Go on an outing to the jungles with this quick fish dish.

- **Day 3**

Breakfast: Fruit and Almond Smoothie

If you think your mornings are excessively occupied for breakfast, reconsider. This smoothie just has four fixings and can be prepared instantly.

Lunch: Veggie and Chicken Pasta Salad

This pasta dish is comparable to lunch for all intents and purposes for supper. Feel free to make a twofold part for extras later in the week.

Supper: Grilled Turkey Burgers

Burgers truly can be solid and delectable. Balance the feast with stove-roasted yam fries for an at-home drive-through dinner.

- **Day 4**

Breakfast: Veggie and Goat Cheese Scramble

Assuming that your taste buds hunger for something appetizing toward the beginning of the day, this veggie and egg scramble is for you. Sautéed peppers, tomatoes, and onions are joined with eggs and cheddar for an inviting and full breakfast plate.

Lunch: Curried Chicken Salad Stuffed Pitas

What separates this chicken sandwich is the velvety Greek yogurt and mayo spread.

Supper: Jamaican Pork Tenderloin with Lemony Green Beans

This fast, basic supper is adequate for summer engagement. Serve it with earthy-colored rice or pilaf for a full feast.

- **Day 5**

Breakfast: Granola with Nuts, Seeds, and Dried Fruit

Lunch: Quinoa Tabbouleh Salad

Quinoa is normally without gluten and is one of the main plant food varieties that is likewise viewed as a total protein. Vegans and meat-eaters alike can partake in this Arabian-motivated salad.

Supper: Beef and Rice Stuffed Peppers

Stuffed peppers are a refined yet family-accommodating choice for any evening of the week.

Make this granola toward the end of the week and piece it out for an entire week of breakfast for yourself as well as your loved ones.

Note: This recipe has a high carb count as a result of the dried organic product. You can change this by eliminating the dried natural product.

- **Day 6**

Breakfast: Banana-Carrot and Pecan Muffins

Serve these biscuits at your next early lunch and you're nearly ensured to have everybody asking for the recipe! The best part is that you can feel much better about eating them as well.

Lunch: Lemony Hummus

Locally acquired hummus can be pungent and flavorless. By making your own, you have some control over the sodium and alter the flavoring however you would prefer.

Supper: Chicken Tortilla Soup

Got extra cooked chicken? Go through it in this hot soup that is certain to fulfill!

- **Day 7**

Breakfast: Tomato and Basil Frittata

Frittatas are an incredible method for spending extra fixings. Present with entire grain toast and cut natural product for a total end-of-the-week breakfast.

Lunch: Butternut Squash and Carrot Soup

Attempt this soup and there's an opportunity you'll at no point ever return to canned assortments in the future.

Supper: Grilled Shrimp Skewers

Shrimp just requires a couple of moments to cook, and that implies when they hit the barbecue, it's dinnertime!

www.ingramcontent.com/pod-product-compliance
Lightning Source LLC
LaVergne TN
LVHW050317160826
845677LV00014B/3438
* 9 7 9 8 8 4 7 9 8 2 4 6 7 *